Kundalini Visions

Empowerment with Kundalini Reiki

By

Kala Maitri

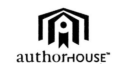

authorHOUSE™

1663 LIBERTY DRIVE, SUITE 200
BLOOMINGTON, INDIANA 47403
(800) 839-8640
WWW.AUTHORHOUSE.COM

First published by AuthorHouse 10/12/04

ISBN: 1-4184-9753-3 (sc)

Printed in the United States of America
Bloomington, Indiana

This book is printed on acid-free paper.

Disclaimer

The material in this book is a general guide for assisting your efforts in for holistic well being. It is not a replacement for traditional health care, medical diagnosis, or medical treatment for illness. Refer to a licensed medical practitioner for medical care. In the event that you use this information in the book for yourself, that is your right, the author does not assume any responsibility for your actions or outcomes.

Acknowledgements

Portions of this text are based on the freely distributed Kundalini Reiki Level One through Three Manuals presumably written by Ole Gabrielson

Cover Artwork

The graphic design, **Kundalini Flow** is by Kala Maitri, who uses intuition within computer generated art to illustrate the primal energy that embodies Kundalini Reiki. Kundalini is a simple but very powerful coiled stream of light that unfolds to touch every facet of one's being. Kundalini Reiki attunements provide the impetus for spiritual rebirth and healing evolvement.

Meditation

Baptisma Etherium

Here we all are now. Standing together in our circle
Closing our eyes. Taking some deep cleansing breaths
Through the nose. Out the mouth

We plant out feet firmly. On the ego continuum
This imaginary line. Beginning a slow, penduluming
movement

Side to side. Black to white. Wrong to right.
Slower, slower, slower. Shedding the lies.

Stopping slowly and finding gray. Imagining the Gray all
around.
Thick and misty. Slowly reaching toward the ground.

We scoop up a portion of this gray. And bringing it slowly
up.
In our hands. Up the midline.
From root too sacral. Slowly to solar plexus.

We feel our hands. Full springy to the touch.
At heart level. Soaring farther free. To our throats
ascending.

A scent of promise. Beyond judgement now.
The depth of soul detachment. As our hands reach our
mind's eye.

We envision a light. Sparked by our movement.
An expanding consciousness. Polishing the Grey.

As we reach above our crown. A myriad of colors mix.
We release this liquid silk. Pausing now.

Breathing in the Essence.
PURE. SOUL. ALIVE.
Embracing the Divine.

Hands dropping slowly. Back to our sides.
Coming back to the room. Free in mind.
Yet, gently listening. With open hearts.

When you feel ready. Okay. Opening our eyes.
Moving our hands and feet around.
Back-> Stretching->Grounding So It Is In Love and Light.

Table of Contents

Description

Kundalini Visions: Empowerment with Kundalini Reiki

Kundalini is a simple but very powerful coiled stream of light that unfolds to touch every facet of one's being. Kundalini Reiki is a healing system through attunements that provides the impetus for spiritual rebirth and healing evolvement. This book is based on the visual imagery received by Kala Maitri, a Kundalini Reiki Master during her classes. It contains a narrative of her journey with the energy. Explaining how to use and teach Kundalini Reiki in the reality of everyday life, this book also shares the empowerment journeys of Vital Earth Energy, Waves of the Mother, and Diamond Energy Completion. It will inspire and bring tears of gratitude!

Chapter 1

Evolving
With
Kundalini

This spiritual journey began somewhat reluctantly with many stops and starts. However, it felt divinely guided that Kundalini Reiki came into my life especially right after the birth of my child, Katrena Violet. As a psychiatric nurse and an intuitive healer I was firmly grounded in reality with many day to day responsibilities including a new infant and a nursing job within a traditional medical setting. I had learned to be in reality while maintaining a firm foot in the other world of the higher dimensions and intuitive spirituality. I had learned to trust my guidance and inner knowing through much education and life experience.

The trauma of my daughter's birth left my body feeling as if I had been crucified and battered. After 24 hours of labor, I had to be cut open while awake to deliver the baby by C-section. It was a very rough transition for her and for me. She cried for the first 24 hours and I was so weak I could barely hold her. I needed major healing. Checking in with my guidance, I clearly intuited, "study Reiki". I felt this was a bit off as I had completed my Usui Reiki Master last June in 2001. What was I supposed to do?

Each night, I meditated before falling into a very much-needed sleep and had the same re-occurring image. There were hundreds of golden symbols coming into my crown chakra. Meditating on the steady strong guidance, I found with great delight that was there more than one Reiki system of healing. I gratefully began to take these attunements by distance and found that with each one I was feeling more and more alive and energized.

I was drawn to the name Kundalini Reiki as I had read every book on Kundalini energy I could get my hands on in the past. There were always warnings about the energy and how one needed to safely use it. Being an earth sign of Taurus though I felt an affinity to anything that was earth-based. So it was without hesitation that I signed up for this course and received my first attunement.

The level one attunement was a very sacred experience because I felt the earth energy come in and enliven my spine and awaken my hand chakras. Immediately, I felt warm and comforted as if I belonged here on earth and was going to be whole once again. I noticed that when I awoke in the morning I was beginning to have a cleanse. There were no other symptoms except for a rather high fever of 102 degrees. My daughter also had this.

At first I did not attribute the fever to the attunement but we both were fine except for the heat. I called the pediatrician as any new mom would for a 3-month-old and began to give her Tylenol. The heat was comforting and I asked to slow the attunement and make it more gentle. The fever did not stop. So I asked my guidance what the fever was for. I received a knowingness that a virus was being burned off from my body to never return again. This would give me great health as I had been slowed down with the Epstein Barr/chronic fatigue syndrome for years. I was grateful that my daughter would also be receiving this healing.

The fever left but the connection to the energy grew and grew. I began to collect the different Reiki Healing systems. For as many in this society believe that "more is better", so I would sign up and receive attunements to a total of 9 systems of healing within a 6 month period. It felt as if I needed the energy to continue living within the dense existence of life. It felt as if my soul had been starved and was now getting real sustenance.

When my Kundalini Reiki master checked in with me to give me level 2 I had not even read the book all the way through. I had felt the details were not so important as the higher vibrating energy coming into my fields providing me with more light and love. I told him that I was just intending Reiki and was hoping that all the different systems of Reiki frequencies would just come through me and that would be enough.

I had missed the point, in my haste to collect with the ego in full force. By hurrying, I had missed the subtle nuances and frequencies. In further meditation, I found that mastery of the Reiki system means one is following the directives and general wishes of the guide that is given for each system. With Kundalini Reiki that meant working in partnership with ascended master Kuthumi.

I began to call in Kuthumi to join what is known as a Healing team, an intended group of beings of light called to help my soul development. I found that Kuthumi was a wonderful teacher, straight and to the point. His influence was usually very subtle but my voice and mannerisms would change through the use of the Kundalini Reiki. The biggest change was the inability to lie or change truth. I became rather startlingly direct and to the point always filled with great love.

3

The level two attunement was also rather dramatic as I remembered placing my hands together in prayer position and activating the energy and huge etheric flames shot up and out of my conjoined hands. The Kundalini flame has been lit.

The level three attunement allowed the energy to go all the way up the main energy channel and out the top of the crown. This attunement provided great relief, as it was a completion of the Kundalini Reiki. During this time I also had my first Kundalini activation. It felt as if a state of pure bliss and oneness following a yoga class. It was as if I was floating in beautiful colors and lights. All my cells were seemingly expanded and for a period of time all I knew was a great and abiding love from the Divine.

As my love for the energies grew I felt that I needed to share these great systems of Reiki. I meditated and was told to be a Reiki teacher. So, I set about buying advertisements and creating brochures presenting the attunements in a menu type fashion. Surely everyone would want to know about these different kinds of Reiki. Surely, I would be able to just teach Reiki and stop all other means of employment.

Here is where I found another truth. Spirit asks for small steps made with great love. Taking one's light out into the world means that you are supported for your contribution that is made in only in Divine will. So, no one signed up for any other Reiki course except for the Kundalini Reiki classes as I was only called to teach my part.

My first class was one student. I had no idea what I was going to do for the 3 hours we were to spend together. The booklet was quite small. I tried to add material and that would not happen. "It is enough," was the guidance I experienced. So, here I was quite apprehensive clutching my booklet for the first class.

Something wonderful happened that class only after I surrendered to the Divine. As I spoke I could feel Kuthumi seemingly speaking through me. My voice changed and the words of pure wisdom and light flowed out of me. The 3 hours went by in a moment. I saw and felt for the first time the depth and strength of the Kundalini Reiki energy. It was as if the frequencies vivified and came through all intuitive channels full force.

My jaw was very tired from channeling. I felt a great heat move through me the entire 3 hours. Going home that evening I marveled about how I was living an ordinary existence one moment and then was transported to a higher plane the next. It was a great miracle.

The students continued to sign up one at a time. Soon there were groups. More opportunities presented themselves for me to teach and share. Each class was just as much for the student as for me. The steam of light and love from earth grew and grew.

I am grateful to share with you in this book my visual perception or artistic interpretation of Kundalini Reiki. There are certainly other ways and means to transport the energies. Please read the words and feel the energy behind the words. There is much light being transmitted within.

Love and Light,
Kala Maitri
September 11th, 2003
Los Gatos, California

Chapter 2

Description
of
Level One

Kundalini Reiki Level One is the beginning of a powerful energy clearing and journey of self-exploration. As one receives the first attunement, the more masculine and active form of the energy is imbued within the energy field of the student. Provided the student to able or willing to identify, clear, and release issues within their energy field, more light is added and the shadow is exposed to light, making the energy field less dense and dark.

This is first and foremost a self-development system, meaning that one is invited to focus on clearing primary issues away, before going out to heal the world. Most healers are inclined to practice their newly used skills and re-ignited energy on everyone except themselves. This why as a teacher, I am often asked by Spirit to tell the student to only practice using this system of Reiki on themselves for thirty days then they are free to heal as called. By dwelling on the self for thirty days, a stable structure and patterning of the energies can be held within one's system.

This form of Reiki is intended to work as a stabilizer on the core chakras: first, second and third centers. It is a building of a pyramid of energy that is the goal for Kundalini Reiki. This pyramid demonstrates that the core energy is strong and provides a base to anchor the higher planetary energies that are coming into the crown chakra. The celestial planetary, cosmic and extraterrestrial energies are to be gathered up and anchored to the earth and below.

Often very spiritual people are visually top heavy with large amounts of higher energies situated in the top three chakras (imagine an inverted pyramid here). The energy stays there not being integrated and could cause some difficulty as the energetic focus in one's life shifts to the higher realms and not on everyday reality. One can escape life responsibilities and issues feeling wonderful for brief sojourns of time. Then the physical beingness of earth is often neglected causing blocks in abundance, vitality, and just the details of living. If your body is out of shape or your diet is poor those are key indicators of this phenomenon.

Know that in order to cultivate one's ability to bring the higher dimensions down to earth practicality, common sense, and earth affinity is important. This is where Kundalini Reiki begins to serve the individual. The first attunement changes some of the energetic structuring of the chakra system. The main energy channel or sushumna is widened to a larger diameter.

The diameter prior to attunement can be visualized sometimes as small as a drinking straw. If the Kundalini flame were to spontaneously arise within this small diameter (also possibly occluded by knots and blocks) there would be nowhere for the energy to rise. It would simply bombard and move in an erratic frantic fashion through out the body seeking an outlet. This condition would describe the imbalanced spiritual awakening with the side effects of Kundalini one often is cautioned about in spiritual texts and traditions.

During the level one attunement the main energy channel is widened and cleared sufficiently so that if the Kundalini flame were to spontaneously ignite, there would be plenty of room for it to rise without an obstruction or impedance. This is one of the main reasons that Kundalini Reiki is the antidote to improper Kundalini awakening.

In level one the Kundalini flame is not lit or activated. This is due to the careful preparation that a student should be told to undertake to ready themselves for level two. Many of the energetic obstructions (called knots and blocks) in the main energy channel are cleared. A sort of energetic plug is kept at the bottom of the first chakra to hold the flame at bay. This does not mean that the student should avoid first chakra issues. Rather any issue as soon as it comes up is meant to cleansed away using the Reiki energy.

The chakras are also scanned during the attunement to see if they need to be adjusted in diameter as well. I visualize the chakras as poker chips stacked one on top of the other. Of course they are really facing out from the body, but this is how I intuit them. Often several chakras can be under or over developed in diameter and flow. This is carefully adjusted so the bottom three chakras are solid and flowing clockwise in the same speed and diameter. Often the diameter after the adjustments are made will go to the edges of the physical body.

Then the heart chakra is gently called upon to enlarge over the thirty-day period to a diameter three times the size of normal. It goes out as wide as your hands can fully extend with arms stretched out by one's sides. This allows for more heart energy to begin to flow. Also this widening sets the stage for the concept of the one unified chakra.

The top three chakras are not so much of a focus during this level but there can be adjustments or comments regarding their issues or developments as well. If the any chakra is closed down or damaged repair work is completed. If the main gift of the chakra is not being used then that is re-ignited. Often there are comments regarding the type of guides and energetic assistance available to help the chakra develop in a balanced way. An example of this would be an intuition of a power animal at the third eye to help with the development of intuition. Hand chakras are opened and cleared during the attunement process as well.

The level one energy itself is very gentle and grounding earth energy. I would describe it as a gentle electric vibration felt especially around the spine and hands. It is more active in its form or rate of vibration and thus gets the designation as being masculine in nature. It is a very deep cleansing energy. The use of the Level one key phrase "Reiki" provides the student with an etheric connection with this energy by intention alone.

If you could imagine for a moment that the word Reiki as you pronounce it is encoded into a language of light and then causes one to be connected with a response of energy. This energetic response is initiated within a grid deeply contained below the earth, in the core or heart of mother earth. The light frequency responds to the request with just the right amount of energy as is needed at a time. It is a very complex process to fathom by our human mind but is simple in the spiritual realms.

In the level one attunement process as I visualize it, there are two specific frequencies that are connected permanently within the student's field. The first is the crystalline core energy and then the lava fire energy. Both are contained in the core and heart of mother earth. I will see multiple strands of lava and crystalline light rise up from the core of earth through all layers of earth and self. They are anchored at the Earth Star chakras. The lava energy allows the purification of the student's path. Crystalline energy is expansive and infuses higher and higher frequencies from earth into the fields.

There are no symbols needed in Kundalini Reiki but it is the connection to the energy one is required to have via the attunement process by a Kundalini Reiki Master Teacher. The teacher is also the channel for the teachings of this system, which are very simple on paper but then more in-depth as an oral tradition. Some students may not receive any oral teachings but that does not mean that the information was never given. All is transmitted to Higher Self that is needed during the attunement process.

Often bits of wisdom are given through the teacher to the student when they are reviewing the text together or going over the oral teachings. Each person has different energetic needs and karmic issues that they will be clearing, so the intention is for the teacher to read the student's energy or chakras and then share what is needed if anything to help with the spiritual journey. Caution is needed here so that the teacher does not take too much responsibility for the student's process. If there are too many questions often it is a sign for the student to be encouraged to the process of self-inquiry and meditation.

If the teacher is conducting a class for more than one student, the energy fields of the students are all merged into one large field. The teacher then reads and attunes the one energy field intending that individual messages are given and received to the intended parties. I have been known to designate the message to pointing to the recipient or being direct if needed in the group setting. Often the students only take in what resonates deeply and leave the rest behind. I do ask that anything that meets with an annoying response is written down to be studied later as it is most likely a meaningful lesson.

Often the energy behind the words is the most important transmission rather than the words themselves. This takes a bit of pressure off a teacher who is not familiar to channeling or intuitive reading. When a class is done by distance I often find more guidance rather then less. To connect with a student by distance and send attunements is just as powerful and effective as in person classes. I choose to tape the readings and spend time with distance students to give them an idea about how sacred and vivid this energy system is.

The main focus of the Kundalini Reiki energies is toward healing the physical and mental processes along with a connection to the guidance of ascended master Kuthumi. Kuthumi is a wise being of light whom functions as a spiritual and psychological teacher. He also has an etheric temple of light in the form of a great crystalline pyramid designed to bring great wisdom and insight to all who journey there. One can also receive initiations into great mysteries and meet Kuthumi asking him for his wisdom as oracle.

I try to describe an ascended master to those students who have never heard that term before as similar to being a saint in the Catholic Church. He has lived on earth before his physical death and now his soul lives on to get closer and closer to Spirit through spiritual service to the inhabitants of earth. So he benefits with spiritual reward when we ask for his assistance. We are not praying to him, but allowing him to be an intermediary between Spirit and us (through him). Often he may be dispatched to come to our aid when we directly send request to Spirit anyway or he will direct the correct form of assistance if it is not in his realm of expertise.

Kuthumi is a master motivator and counselor. He is very straight and to the point. He encourages action and enthusiasm. Spiritual people may collect great healing and knowledge for themselves. Kuthumi often asks one to integrate the knowledge into the physical realm in very unique and wonderful ways allowing you to take your unique talent or mission out into the world and become part of the world solution.

Although I have never corresponded with Ole Gabrielsen, I am grateful for his connection with Kuthumi and establishing this system of Reiki. He is from Denmark and is a meditation master there. He spent time in direct presence or communion with Kuthumi who bestowed to him the Kundalini Reiki system.

The five techniques contained in level one are there for everyday practical use. In order to progress in clearing and strengthening the energy field, one should practice and commit the techniques to memory. A careful review of each technique is done during the teaching portion of the class. I advise reading the text through at least seven different times in the 30 day period.

1. Laying on of Hands

One can do a self healing by placing a hand or hands anywhere on the body and intending to connect with the energy using the key phrase Reiki. The energy will flow in and go where it is needed. A full treatment is completed in 3-5 minutes. Using the energy anytime when it is needed is recommended. Frequency and consistency of treatment is always a clear message by Kuthumi. Often our issues have layers like an onion and need the repetition to really see progress.

This method would also work with healing others. Place your hands where guided while being in a centered, sacred place. Remembering to breathe and ground yourself to earth. Then think or say the key phrase Reiki. Stop when the energy ceases or feels complete.

Know that the shoulders are a special point of power and stability within this Reiki system. So to start a healing on someone you could go to the shoulders and run the energy for 3-5 minutes. I often see this as an opener to bring things up to the surface that are then released in a gentle and cleansing manner. There is no need to do any formal hand placement or sequence with the healing. Often, I will travel to places where I see things or sense things but one hand placement is certainly effective.

2. Distance Prayer

The first name is the energetic signature of a being. That is all one needs to access a friend, client or student for a distance healing. I am often guided to say to students, " This is how Jesus prayed" when describing this technique. It is enough to ask someone permission to do a Reiki healing by saying "Can I say a prayer for you?"

You write the person's first name with the pointer finger of one hand into the palm chakra of other hand while intending to connect to their essence or Higher self. Then placing the hand chakras together begin running the energy. This prayer position is the masculine form of action of prayer. It is allowing the person to be surrounded and enfolded in light for their highest good and healing.

I did not want to be walking around in daily life with my hands in prayer position. So, I asked Spirit, "How can I do this so I can clear at work or make it more functional?" The answer I received was to hold my hand chakras together with the fingers on the opposite wrists. I was told this was the feminine receptive mudra. That it would clear very gently and effectively as well.

After several months I found a beautiful book called Healing Mudras by Sabrina Mesko, that contained this very hand position. It also helped all the chakras in five minutes and helped to bring one-pointed attention. Now I could walk down the hallway at work or in the grocery store while clearing issues as soon as I was aware of them.

13

3. Clearing Space

Just as our body contains issues to be cleared so may our etheric space. In our home and work environment there may need to be some spiritual clearing. I view this technique as etheric saging minus the cough producing smoke. Write in the palm of one hand, "my home" or the name of the location. Then place the hand chakras together running the energy with the key phrase Reiki. Please use this technique if there is a lot of arguing or stress going on in the home or office. It can be used as a supplement to calling in the angels or saging with real sage.

#4. Relationship Tending

This is one of the most powerful techniques of this level. There are cords generated each time we think or talk to someone. Any interaction can send a spider-web like connection to the other party. If the cord is not cleared over time it will be larger in diameter and begin to drain one's energy. Often there may not be just unconditional love flowing back and forth.

One can be sending these cords without even being conscious of their occurrence. One can receive these cords without being aware of the source. Often, a cording has occurred if a person's name suddenly pops into your head. They can be thinking about you and then it happens. Regardless of how it happens, it is your responsibility to clear these cords and keep your side of the relationship clear.

If two people represented by my two hands side by side with each as a ball of light are vibrating at the same frequency and sending cords to each other suddenly get into a denser frequency, it is imperative that you move up to the heart with forgiveness and love. To do this allows you to take care of your side and be free from the cords. Your hand or ball of light would rise up higher.

Now it is not in your power to move the other party up to the heart or higher in frequency. They have to deal with their own karma. They can however choose to follow your lead and rise up to your level. Or they will try to cord you but you are higher and not going to be pulled down. Sometimes this technique causes a gentle release of the other person to the background or out of your life. Sometimes the other person may forget why they were upset and the relationship carries on in harmony. There are very many scenarios. You are practicing good spiritual boundaries by not manipulating their energy and focusing on your responsibility.

To activate this technique, write into your hand chakra the following phrase: *"my relationship with_____"*. You can also clear the cords for another person's relationship if given permission such as healer-client role. Then you would write, *"_____'s relationship with their mother"*. Allow the energy to flow with the key phrase and stop when the energy stops.

5. Goals and Issues

This technique is one of the more fun ways to work with energy. If you are a goal-oriented person and have a lot to accomplish you need to make sure your goal is based in Divine Will. Often when the goal is an ego-oriented goal, then there will be a lot of struggle, doubt, and spinning of one's wheels. To make sure you are in Divine will, write the words of the goal in the palm of your hand and then run the energy. This allows for the goal to placed inside the Tap Root chakra and supported the by light. If it is in Divine will the goal will flourish and flower coming up in your awareness when action is needed. If the goal is not for the highest good, you will be able to release your attachment to it much with much ease. You will not be upset when letting go and will be able to move forward to the next great thing. So for example, some goals to activate might be, "my book" "new car" "abundance".

When you become aware of an issue arising in your life, immediately write the phrase of what it might be. Then run the energy to cleanse it out. However this Reiki is filled with common sense. For instance, if you were to have a broken leg you could take a moment to run the energy but then ask what to do about it. Getting to a doctor to get the bone set would be the next common sense direction. Sometimes spiritual people disqualify the obvious looking for a miracle when common sense and the next step is all that is needed. Some issues are instantly transmuted in the light as well.

Level one contains the most techniques and ways to work with the energy. There are also individualized attunements given to you from Kuthumi through your teacher. Please practice these attunements as needed with the instructions that are given. Often your teacher is guided to connect with the attributes needed to either speed or stabilize your soul development. Take notes and enjoy the attunements as an opportunity to be connected with great light.

If the attunement causes a cleanse which are symptoms that a lot of density is being transmuted and cleared, please ask Spirit to slow down the attunement process. Also you can ask your Healing team for guidance as to what is happening and the reasons for the symptoms. Any healing crisis is an opportunity to clear out ancient wounds and issues. If in doubt on what to do, contact your teacher.

Please note that since the planetary energies are speeded up most of the cautions and limitations are not applicable any more within the original text of the Kundalini Reiki Manuals. Please use wisdom, creativity and discernment with the energy and trust your guidance as you integrate the practice of Kundalini Reiki into your life.

This ends the description of level one. If you are a teacher please refer to the chapter on Class Organization for further instruction.

Chapter 3

Description
of
Level Two

Kundalini Reiki Level Two is a continuation of the Kundalini energetic spectrum but the vibration shifts to a more feminine receptive mode. The earth energy is perceived as increasingly nurturing, soothing and gentle. Often the energy comes in waves from the core of earth in pulsation as if to experience the heart beat or rhythm of mother earth. It is a sacred time of thirty days to move deep within your being and gently bring yourself respite, mercy and deep healing.

The attunement in this level is the most important portion of the class as it continues to stabilize and transform the core energies of the first, second, and third chakras. The Kundalini flame is ignited during the attunement and begins to rise slowly in the lower three chakras. The flame only ascends up the main energy channel to rest at the top of the solar plexus. The actual flame may be quite small initially for some but fuller for others. The way to get the flame strong and clear is to practice the Kundalini Reiki meditation given by the teacher.

There is a new key phrase to connect with this specific energy. One would center, ground and say or intent "Kundalini Reiki" This phrase again is translated to the language of light and is connected to a grid deep within the core of the earth. A possible description of this key phrase is that it surrounds whatever is intended in light. There it is transmuted, transformed or additional common sense guidance is given to resolve the issue. An instant transmutation would look like the energy of the issue being dissolved and then recycled back to original essence. Perhaps the image of a star exploding and then being reabsorbed by the atmosphere would be an analogy.

If there is more than one layer or additional guidance is needed to transmute the issue, please check in with Spirit or the Healing team. Every issue is resolved exactly at the right time and space in Divine Will. With careful meditation one can sit with the issue and then call in Spirit dialoguing with the how to clear and what needs to be done. Some issues are karmic in nature and the lesson of working with them is the healing itself. So please enjoy the process of raising your vibration by surrounding issues with light.

The powerful, divine meditation given in this level is activated either in a sitting or reclining pose. One connects with the energy by centering and then either by intending or speaking the key phrase, "Kundalini Reiki Meditation". This starts an energetic process about five minutes in length that cleanses and realigns the chakras.

Each time the Kundalini flame is enlightened and strengthened. My perception of this meditation is that it re-centers you in the core of the first, second, and third chakras, while preparing the energetic pyramid. It also clears the burden of reactivity allowing one to discern truth and stay centered. One can use this meditation as often as needed per day.

In the attunement process for level two, I was guided to connect the students to an energy source from mother earth called the Waves of the Mother. To describe this is an energy wave that contains very gentle pulsation that comes at intervals in waves. It feels wonderfully cleansing and powerful to raise this energy, but one has to be connected to it through the level two attunement.

Sit or stand firmly grounded into the earth by whatever grounding mechanism you are most familiar with. Center in your heart and feel your heart beat with great love. Now focus on as you raise your hands our at your side palms facing up. Begin to gently lower and raise the hands stating or intending the key phrase, Waves of the Mother. Feel the energy shift and come in from the earth up through your energy fields. Continue to summon the energy as you either push the energy out with palms facing out in front of your chest toward an intended focal point.

Let's use the globe of earth as a visualization. See the energy going to surround and enfold the earth with healing vibrations. Continue to push the energy until it feels complete. You can also send the energy to any space or place within your own fields. Move the palms facing inward and pull the energy of the Waves of the Mother toward your own heart. Feel the strong current of Unconditional Love from your Divine Mother. Know that each time you feel alone this will bring you great strength on your path.

The attunement process also yields another important energy shift for level two, the activation of DNA. Visualizing the two main frequencies, the crystalline and lava energies rising up from the core of mother earth in very wide beams of light. They enter the individual's energy field at the moment of self and rise through the main energy channel through all the simultaneous past lifetimes, through the

19

chakra system and out the crown up all levels or dimensions of self to Spirit.

These two spirals are connected to grids and light structures, effectively plugged in and turned on if that is for the highest good. Some students are ready for all strands of DNA to be activated and brought on line as others are only in the infant stages of healing and less is activated.

By meditating on the corresponding DNA Activation Attunement one can take the next steps to learning how to work with this ancient code. One may be guided to learn about the family tree or genetic heritage of relatives and elders. It is important to clear the DNA back to original essence. One might be guided to study DNA with classes, books, or music.

There are also other individualized attunements given to you from Kuthumi through your teacher. Please practice these attunements as needed with the instructions that are given. Take notes and enjoy the attunements as an opportunity to be connected with great light.

Often your teacher is guided to connect the student to feminine attributes of energy that are needed to become whole. For some students who have disowned the power of feminine heritage it will expand your concept of the Divine Energies of Spirit. Go gently with yourself if you had not previously reclaimed the Mother energy as sacred. Mother energy is key to becoming abundant and successful in reality on the earth plans.

If the attunement causes any cleansing which are symptoms that a lot of density is being transmuted and cleared, please ask Spirit to slow down the attunement process. Also you can ask your Healing team for guidance as to what is happening and the reasons for the symptoms. Any healing crisis is an opportunity to clear out ancient wounds and issues. If in doubt on what to do, contact your teacher.

Please note that since the planetary energies are speeded up most of the cautions and limitations are not applicable any more within the original text of the Kundalini Reiki Manuals. Please use wisdom, creativity and discernment with the energy and trust your guidance as you integrate the practice of Kundalini Reiki into your life.

This ends the description of level two. If you are a teacher please refer to the chapter on Class Organization for further instruction.

Chapter 4

Description
of
Level Three

Kundalini Reiki Level Three is the completion of the Kundalini Reiki series. Know that there is a great energy release whenever a process reaches a full circle. Imagine it as having open windows or programs on the computer. When you finish level three you can close the window and have more energy available for other parts of your life. It is a Divine celebration to receive the final attunement in this series and be designated as a Kundalini Reiki Master.

In level three there is not so much emphasis on clearing the main energy channel, chakra clearing, or intuitive reading by the teacher. If the student has been diligent they will be prepared for this attunement with a clearly widened and unblocked channel. The issues that have arisen in the last 60 days have hopefully allowed the student opportunity to raise their vibration through cleansing and surrounding in the light with the two key phrases, Reiki and Kundalini Reiki.

One continues to use both key phrases, all of the techniques, individualized attunements, and other intuitions regularly and great patience through one's lifetime. The energy field is transformed to allow massive amounts of wonderful energy to sustain the student in everyday life with plenty of vitality, abundance, groundedness, and support.

Kundalini energy is purified and true. It can be described as primordial earth energy that embodies Kundalini Reiki. Kundalini is described in this Reiki as a simple but very powerful coiled stream of light that unfolds to touch every facet of one's being. The series of attunements hopefully have provided the impetus for spiritual rebirth and healing evolvement.

There is a self-inquiry that one has to undergo with taking each level of this Reiki. Am I ready to take the attunement? Have I practiced the techniques and learned? Am I clearing and asking for guidance daily and as needed? Am I intending to be part of the solution for earth and all whose lives I touch? Am I holding the higher the vibrations of light within my heart? Am I intending for the highest good and healing? Is my life centered on Divine Will? Have I cleared a percentage of my karma and now can move upward to the next level? Am I following the next steps of guidance without trying to rush to the outcome?

When there is a certainty that level three is to be called in, know that this level is another chance to do intense clearing. I ask that all students commit to the following Reiki healing sequence for 30 days (at least) after receiving the master level attunement. The purpose for this is to really anchor these energetic frequencies into your existence or essence.

The Reiki healing sequence is a list of all the key phrases from level one to level three done as a healing discipline sometime throughout the day. There are several options to accomplish this. One can wake up first thing in the morning with a list by the bedside and run the energies for several minutes with each key phrase. The simple hands on healing method is used.

Alternately, one can ask that the Healing Team or angelic realm perform this sequence at night before going to sleep. Simply center, state the intention and list the key phrases. It may go something like this:

"I ask that my angels or Healing Team run the Reiki healing sequence for two hours as I sleep providing me with a gentle energy clearing and integration. I ask for the following sequence of frequencies one at a time until it is complete for my highest good and healing":

Reiki
Kundalini Reiki
Diamond Reiki
Crystalline Reiki
DNA Reiki
Birth Trauma Reiki
Location Reiki
Past Life Reiki

There is also the chance to run the energy if one commutes in the car and can still drive safely. Use your discretion and common sense here. I have the key phrases taped on the dash of the car and at a light will place my hand on my body and run the energy. The goal is to incorporate the energy in everyday living interweaving the frequencies to uplift your life.

In Kundalini Reiki Three all the previous attunements and processes are reinforced energetically. This means includes all the energetic restructuring and individualized attunements are accelerated and adjusted to a higher frequency.

The higher energy bodies are especially cleared as the full Kundalini Flame arises and goes up the remainder of the main energy channel and out of the crown chakra. The extra attunements are connected with the key phrases to the grids of light. I will now explain each key phrase and delineate some important guidance to maximize your experience.

Diamond Reiki is a powerful expansive energy. It is primarily used during meditation to infuse the power of the soul of earth into the energy fields. It enlightens and brings alive all energies increasing and accelerating their power and ability. Kuthumi places an etheric diamond in the crown chakra as a gift that naturally amplifies energy. It is a blessed gift that symbolizes your ongoing commitment to the union of heaven and earth through light work. It can of course be refused or accepted at will. To activate this key phrase, center and say or intend, "Diamond Reiki".

Crystalline Reiki is a powerful root cause clearing technique that dissolves crystal formations in any dimension, chakra, or part of the body that needs to be released. A crystal is formed that holds the memory or trauma of any damage that is unresolved. Often these are ancient memories, but can be as simple a skinned knee from childhood. In the original manual it states that hands on method is the only to use this key phrase. Use your guidance regarding this. I found that several treatments might be needed to clear and dissolve the crystalline structure completely. To activate this key phrase, center and say or intend, "Crystalline Reiki".

DNA Reiki is a wonderful chance to work further on activating and clearing the DNA blueprint. As you collect the family, genetic and past-life information to be cleared, use the DNA Reiki key phrase to transmute out these issues. I found that if you use of instance the issue "breast cancer" and write it in the palm of the hands then run the DNA Reiki, it can be quite profound and clearing. You can use the hands on method as well. To activate this key phrase, center and say or intend, "DNA Reiki".

It takes time and dedication to access and identify what needs to be cleared. Often the male holds the work of clearing the genetic lineage seven generations behind and ahead. If you are a woman, you can still do this work but talk to a male elder of the light on your Healing team who holds the seed encodements for your blueprint. Remember that you do need to replace or rewrite any code, gene, or sequence that you clear. I like to intend that the Beloved I AM to be infused into the places and spaces that were released for your highest good and healing.

Birth Trauma Reiki is one of the most highly needed frequencies on the planet for women and children to be freed. As I meditated on this key phrase, the birth issues and giving birth issues were the focus to clear. Any child who transitions into earth is met with trauma during the birth process. There is in fact, a whole psychological model by Stanislov Grof that describes which portion of the birthing process leads to a resulting psychological dysfunction that can manifest. So it is imperative to clear with the Birth trauma Reiki key phrase. I often see the end result of a complete healing as a powerful bubble of light surrounding the infant as they are born. Birth and rebirth issues on the ascension spiral can also be cleared if one subscribes to the birth, death, and rebirth model of evolvement.

Finally, the mother or anyone who has given birth in any lifetime desperately needs this form of Reiki. Our society does not allow women to voice the wounds of giving birth and tending to the newborn. Women are preconditioned to be silent in order to make it a happy time. The traumas and feelings are suppressed in the female organs. Often times the birthing process and early months of mothering hold very dense vibrations of shame, inadequacy, horror, pain, and other indescribable thoughts and feelings.

If these issues are not cleared there is a double impact. The feminine organs may become diseased to signal their presence and/ or the bond between child and mother can be complicated. The infant can pick up on the heavy emotions and be distant and behaviorally challenged as a result. The use of the Birth Trauma Reiki allows the wounds to be cleared and deep and abiding forgiveness to come in between the child and mother-regardless of age. To activate this key phrase, center and say or intend, "Birth Trauma Reiki".

Location Reiki is similar to the Level One, technique # 4, regarding relationships. Here it is the relationships with physical earth possessions or even the earth itself. When a person gets stuck on a certain form that is no longer in Divine Will, or needs to let go of any old possession to get a new one, or is in hoarding consciousness, this key phrase is the antidote. To activate this key phrase, center and say or intend, "Location Reiki".

There are cords or energetic attachments to our preferences or desires on the physical plane. Some of use may be very attached to "keeping up with the Jones". As a consumer based society we often turn to shopping, or possessing to make our ego based selves feel full. This technique clears away our attachment to certain possessions, habits, or behaviors that weigh us down. Often when you are trying to manifest a new car you might need to write "car" in the palm of your hand and run the Location Reiki on it.

Imagine that we have a worthiness quota in life that we may or may not be aware of. It allows one to hold a certain energetic amount that translates to a dollar amount of possessions on the physical plane at any given time. In truth we are unlimited but most humans have agreed unconsciously to only hold this much worthiness or wealth quantification within space and time.

If we have closets full of clutter this is filling up our quota so not so much new stuff can come in. It may be stuck up in a holding pattern if we have manifested in on the etheric waiting for us to clear out the old. We can of course increase out worthiness quota or simply choose to clear out the old. The Location Reiki will cut the cords to the old and our resistance to making changes based in wisdom, love and power on the physical plane related to abundance and manifesting!

Past Life Reiki clears out any resulting patterns, beliefs, and wounds, lessons that are stubbornly re-occurring because they are based in past life. If you are having the feelings of "Oh not that again" it is most likely a past life issue. To activate this key phrase, center and say or intend, "Past Life Reiki".

I use this Reiki on clients during a healing session to intuit the pictures or snapshots of the past life that are still affecting the present. Past life issues are not meant to become attached to, as they are simply for information only. One may not even need to know what is being cleared. If you are learning about a past life where you were famous and then spend a lot of time and energy around glorifying it, the ego is at its work helping you to miss the point.

If by chance you are meditating on past life and being to experience it in your present day body. Quickly ask for your Healing team to assist and place a silver cord on your body and float above the past life. Visualize what is happening and allow the angels to clear the issue with some minor direction.

Past Lives are simultaneously being lived in another parallel dimension. Intend that this life you are living be the path of the most light. Ask that any wounds are cleared and any gifts or talents are magnetized to the present. One can write "past life gifts" in the palm of the hands and place the hands in prayer position or the feminine mudra running the Reiki. Profound integration and healing divinatory wisdom is available through the use of Past Life Reiki.

Balance is key phrase attached to a hand mudra. It is a wonderful technique to balance all the energetic systems in the body. One simply centers and places all the fingers and thumbs together of both hands while saying or thinking "Balance" Hold this mudra for 30 seconds and breathe allowing the process to get under way. This process takes an hour to complete but you do not have to remain in meditation during this time.

A whole Reiki healing session now can last a complete hour with the use of the different key phrases. Please note that the most powerful clearing and cleansing key phrases are the Reiki and Kundalini Reiki. One should start a healing session with at least one of these and then work through several of the level three key phrases.

Often times I will place my hands on someone and the correct phrase to state will just pop into my head. If it is not clear how to proceed ask your Healing team to clarify or make a really simple for you to know how to proceed. Healing is supposed to be easy and fun as well as healing for you!

You also can now attune objects as Reiki channels with a special key phrase. You will feel guided to infuse the object with the Reiki light. Hold the object that can be anything either in your physical hand or intuitive awareness and say to your Higher self, I *ask that this* _____*(object) may be attuned as a Reiki channel."*

It is common for students to then be asking how the object then helps them out. I prefer to think that after an object is attuned, it provided a clearing that is 3-5 minutes in length or as Spirit intends.

There also may be other individualized attunements given to you from Kuthumi through your teacher. Please practice these attunements as needed with the instructions

29

that are given. Take notes and enjoy the attunements as an opportunity to be connected with great light.

If the master attunement causes any cleansing, which are symptoms that a lot of density is being transmuted and cleared, please ask Spirit to slow down the attunement process. Also you can ask your Healing team for guidance as to what is happening and the reasons for the symptoms. Any healing crisis is an opportunity to clear out ancient wounds and issues. If in doubt on what to do, contact your teacher.

Please note that since the planetary energies are speeded up most of the cautions and limitations are not applicable any more within the original text of the Kundalini Reiki Manuals. Please use wisdom, creativity and discernment with the energy and trust your guidance as you integrate the practice of Kundalini Reiki into your life.

This ends the description of Level Three. As you are now a teacher please refer to the chapter on Class Organization for further instruction in preparing and attuning students.

Chapter 5

Class
Organization

As one moves through the mastery of the techniques and energies, they are often guided to begin attuning others in their life to Kundalini Reiki. Kuthumi usually gives gentle nudges and provides a deep inner knowing when it is time to step into the role of Kundalini Reiki Master Teacher. I believe that Kuthumi confers this designation of Master to those who agreed to teach this system of Reiki. If you are not meant to teach Kundalini Reiki it is still in the best interest to complete coursework to raise the vibration within your system.

One does not need to practice Kundalini Reiki the way I present it. I want to make that very clear that this is my artistic interpretation of the energies and experiences that I perceive. I am in no way claiming to have enhanced or brought any new material to the Kundalini Reiki lineage. I am simply describing what I see so that you can make your own observation. Please take what you like or resonant with and leave the rest. It is presented in the Spirit of Sacred Oneness.

The message I have received continuously since early 2003 during the teaching of this system are that due to the planetary energies becoming accelerated the "rules have been thrown out". Meaning that most of the cautions and limitations are not applicable any more within the original text of the Kundalini Reiki Manuals. Please use wisdom, creativity and discernment with the energy and trust your guidance as you teach the practice of Kundalini Reiki to others.

To pass on attunements to others all that is really needed is the following key phrase: Hold the person you are attuning in your intuitive awareness and say to your Higher self, *I ask that (name) _____ may be attuned in Kundalini Reiki Level (number)_____ "*.

I will now describe in detail how I conduct both an in-person class and a distance class so that one might be inspired to bring out the natural creativity of this energy. Class structure involves three main elements: 1) Review of the written text, 2) Oral tradition or teaching and 3) attunement processes.

Class Outline for In-Person Classes

- Introductions
- Share of Your Story
- Meditation to Set Energies
- Review of Text
- Break
- Questions/Clarifications
- Explanation of the Attunement Process
- Chakra Clearing / Intuitive Reading/Guided Meditation
- Attunement Ceremony
- Questions/ Review

- Closures with Gratitude
- Energy Clearing

Class Outline for Distance Courses

1) Meditation to Set Energies
2) Attunement
3) Review of Text
4) Chakra   Clearing/Intuitive   Reading/   Guided Meditation
5) Closures with Gratitude
6) Energy Clearing
7) Review/Questions by E-mail

Attunement Ceremony

I have been guided to facilitate the attunement process with more ritual if needed.

In a centered and grounded state, stand up and approach the front of the student placing your hands on the crown chakra with an triangle or pyramid shape present between the thumbs and part of the two pointer fingers.

Standing and holding the space for a moment. Ask for permission to give the attunement. When the student states "yes" or you sense this on a Higher self level, continue with the key phrase: *I ask that (name) _____ may be attuned in Kundalini Reiki Level (number)_____ "*.

Sense or visualize the energy coming up from the earth in your body and out through your hands and into the person's crown chakra. It may appear as multiple ribbons of golden energy. This energy then flows quite rapidly down the person's energy field anchoring in the earth.

Breathing and moving your hands to hold the shoulders. Intending to stabilize the attunement in the person's energy. Seeing or visualizing the ribbons of light again travel down anchoring into the earth.

Moving to hold each hand and intending to bless the healer for all the healing work that is to occur for the Highest good on their path. As you hold each hand in sandwich, sense if you need to clear out any old energy. You would do this by lifting out the energy from the palm chakra and discarding it away for the person's energy field.

Then allow or instruct the person to move their hands to prayer position.

Moving down to the feet and holding to the feet as you bless this person as they walk on their path in Kundalini Light. Then sometimes but not always, take a very deep breath and blow up the main energy channel a color, element, or form of healing light you sense the person needs to help clear.

Standing and grounding in front of the person, clearing your energy and putting asking that the attunement to Kundalini Reiki now be complete internally as you discard and clear any unneeded energy by whatever method before moving on to the next person.

This will start an energetic process within the person that lasts about 25 minutes. This process is automatic and nothing you perform or do affects it. That is why only the key phrase to start the attunement is needed.

To provide a distance attunement, the teacher can imagine the student standing or sitting in front of them and then proceed with the attunement steps as if in person.

Prior to completing a Level Three attunement have the student hand scan over the head to feel the difference with or without the fully activated Kundalini flame.

Only attune children over the age of eight. I am told that a cleanse can be handled very efficiently after that age. I choose to attune my daughter at age 2 but she did have quite a cleanse and I would not choose to do that again.

Please free to use the guided meditation script or CD's called Vital Earth Energy (Level One), Waves of the Mother (Level Two) or Diamond Energy Completion (Level Three) as the intuitive reading/chakra clearing part of the class.

Oral teachings are the same as channeling from Higher Source or Kuthumi.

Often times I will observe myself saying the most interesting things during a class. I will say to myself, "Now where did that come from?" Then, I will look at one of the students and see their heart open or tears come down their cheeks. Never discount the importance of anything that is said during a class.

My students often wanted tapes of the class. I would try to tape and reproduce them. It never worked out. That is when the CD idea came through. The CDs hold a very high vibration and healing. They renew the connection to the original attunement and if played on low in the background provide energy clearing as well.

The individualized attunements are a result of guidance when reading the student's energy field. I will be drawn to discuss a certain theme or issue that a person really needs to get to move forward. Often there are similar themes in people. There are attunements that I know everyone would benefit from so everyone gets key phrase to practice. Please allow yourself to seemingly make up attunements when you start teaching. It is a very real process and just requires some confidence and inner knowing.

Always center in your heart and know that Spirit is guiding you to teach from the Heart of Mother Earth. Namaste in Love and Light, Dear Ones.

Chapter 6

Guided
Meditation Scripts

Vital Earth Energy

The intention for this meditation, Vital Earth Energy is to provide the listener each time with gentle, healing energy that expands and opens clearing and cleansing that main energy channel, realigning the chakras, and anchoring into the body this Vital Earth Energy. So allow yourself to listen and know deep within that you are love. You are healed. You are whole.

I call forth from Spirit a beautiful pillar of light descending down from the Source of All There Is into the center of you. This beautiful pillar is a wonderful high frequency white light from Spirit that surrounds you and enclosed you in a beautiful chamber of meditation, healing, and energy expansion. Surrounding this pillar of white light I call forth the planetary and cosmic hierarchy, representatives of the angelic kingdom, the divine ascended masters, the lady masters, your own guardian angel and your guides of the light. I call in the spirit animals and the earth spirits to surround you in a beautiful circle by intention providing you a sacred space.

I call in AA Michael and his band of mercy to surround you and enfold you in his precious cloak of blue light. Removing from you any fear, doubt, density, negativity, guilt, past life karma, old contracts, anything that is no longer for the Highest Good to be gently released on the exhale now. As he takes these issues all the way from your cellular memory down, he brings them up to the heavens for light.

A beautiful shower, a golden mist of Christ Consciousness reigns down upon you. Breathe deeply in this beautiful light and allow yourself to be restored and renewed. Clearing out the old on the exhale. Bringing in Christ Consciousness on the inhale. I ask that each time you listen, speak or read this meditation your vibratory level, your cells, and your entire being is infused with beautiful light of Christ Consciousness. Going to the next level and definitely the next step of your life purpose and journey.

And I call forth AA Michael, AA Uriel, AA Gabriel, and AA Raphael to stand in the four corners of your space while you listen. They send healing transmissions to reawaken your gifts for your life purpose. Allowing then to gently enfold you in beautiful waves of angelic light.

And as your breathe deeply, bring your awareness to a place about 24 " below the earth. This is your beautiful tap root chakra. This is your place of pure potential. Scan this place with your awareness and see if there is anything to be cleared out. We will now ask AA Michael to stand by holding the space. Just surrender anything in this energetic space that is not of your highest potential and nurturing for you. As he takes anything you released to the light, we ask for that space to be infused with beautiful rich, dark, loam, earth energy.

This is your sacred vessel. This is your energetic womb below the earth where you can plant seeds of your projects, life purpose, and desires. Allowing them to be surrendered and to come up in your awareness when they are ready as full flowering as full expressions. And I see here lots of earth spirit energy working with you to manifest all your needs and desires. You deserve to receive in great abundance, in true potential as a child of Spirit. Taking a deep breath and allowing that chakra to spin clockwise.

Moving up the channel, widening the channel, now to an area about 12 " below your feet. This is a place called the Earth Star Chakras. These chakras are actually visualized as mini stars that are platforms holding you very grounded on earth. We ask that these be cleared with a beautiful sapphire light at this time. That they spin clockwise and are anchored to the very core of Mother Earth with two specific vibrations of energy: The crystalline core energy and lava fire energy. Both are contained in the core and heart of mother earth. See multiple strands of lava and crystalline light rise up now from the core of earth through all layers of earth and self anchoring at these platforms. The lava energy makes you walk in fire, in truth, in life, in purification on your path. Crystalline infuses higher and higher frequencies. Accepting and blending with these two energies totally connected to the core of mother earth. Your earth star chakras spinning clockwise.

Moving your attention up the channel and widening it to your actual feel chakras. They are beautiful dark black, the color of true potential. Allowing yourself to see all the colors held within this beautiful darkness, this void. When you walk on your journey you allow yourself to let go and destroy all old forms that hold space that are no longer serving your highest good. You allow yourself to move in cycles with the lunar phases. You allow yourself to be in your power as a man or woman here on earth. Taking a deep breath now. Seeing them spinning clockwise.

Taking a deep breath now moving up the channel widening the channel. Placing your attention on your knee chakras. These are your movement centers see the tan to brown color moving clockwise. Sense if you need to add more movement to your life. High frequency energies are often anchored here on earth through movement and breath. Put your hands on your knees now and think Movement Attunement. This will allow all the sacred energies pouring through your crown chakra to be anchored down in and move in the rhythm of your mind, body, spirit, and emotions. Allowing all your energy bodies to move at just the right time and space continuum. Anytime when you feel you are moving too forward into the future or are too much in the past activate this attunement and know that you are in alignment with Spirit.

Moving up the channel, widening the channel now, going to your root chakra. This is a beautiful place of connection, abundance and security here on earth. Know deep within that you are supported 100% on your life mission. See this chakra, a beautiful ruby color spinning clockwise, allowing yourself to release on the exhale: Any names, limiting beliefs systems, any separations you place internally or externally. Releasing on the exhale. Inhaling and allowing this pure place to be filled with ruby light. This crystalline ruby light mixes with a beautiful garnet light from AA Uriel who wants you to walk in truth, the truth of Divine Abundance and prosperity. Knowing that as you give you will receive. Please given to yourself first and hold yourself in this space.

Building the energy. Taking guided action one step at a time. Connecting in the light. Connecting from the heart. AA Michael at this time cuts all the cords blessing the connections and releasing them with love. And he also wants you to breathe the breath of fire daily building your power in the first chakra in your core in your connection to earth.

Taking a deep breath widening the channel moving up the channel to the sacral chakra, a beautiful orange color.

Allowing you creativity and expression, sacred sexuality and Divine Love. Feel here the unity of male and female. Feel the unity of oneness. Feel here your Unity Attunement by placing both hands on your belly and thinking to yourself Unity Attunement. Healing, becoming one, knowing a beautiful orange color here. Spinning clockwise. All is One.

Taking a deep breath, moving up the channel, widening the channel to your solar plexus chakra. Beautiful sun, solar yellow energy here, spinning clockwise. Now AA Michael commands all ego agendas, attachments, beliefs, plans be surrendered to the light. For it is only the True Divine Will that is to unfold in the perfect space and time within the rhythm of your soul. Taking a deep breath and exhaling the ego. Allowing any negative consciousness to be taken to the light escorted by AA Michael now. Placing your hands on your solar plexus and thinking Divine Will Attunement. Keeping yourself surrounded by angels and asking for help very moment of the day to be guided inspired and in true power, strength of a spiritual warrior.

Taking a deep breath, moving up the channel, widening the channel now to your heart chakra. This heart chakra has been gently moving and opening out about three times the size of its normal dimension. This gentle expansion happens over the next thirty days and to infinity. You allow this beautiful emerald green color to hold you in love and to be love. As you learn to work with this energy, let it go out into the world and hold people in its space. You are truly blessed. You are truly love. Allowing the Christ Consciousness energy to come into this space. Allowing the connection to the Higher Self here. For you are working as a team for your Higher Self and for your soul group or monad. Knowing that love is the only thing that is real. Accepting this blessing and grace from Spirit now. Be filled, be overflowing, be abundant with love. Taking a deep breath now releasing any grief, past relationship issues, struggling to connect with anyone, struggling to be understood. For true love casts out all fear.

Allow yourself to be love. Holding this space for yourself each day and growing in love and light.

Taking a deep breath. Moving up the channel widening the channel to a space behind your sternum. Your soul purpose chakra or high heart chakra. It may be many beautiful colors it may be one. See if you can sense what color your particular chakra is. Allow it to go out in front of your chest straight ahead into the world. Your life purpose is sacred and you know that you do not need to anyone else's job. This creates abundance. So accept that all you have to do is your job, given to you by Spirit at the time of your sacred contract before you came into this world. By meditating on your life purpose or the next step is all Spirit ever asks, besides asking for support from your brothers and sisters of the light, from your higher guidance, from your healing team. You are supported 100% know this, have a confidence that you will evolve spiritually and carry out your highest purpose exactly as it is intended for your Highest Good.

Taking a deep breath, moving up the channel, widening the channel to your beautiful throat chakra. You allow yourself to express yourself in whatever form that takes. Whether that be through movement, thought, art, voice, the written word, computer, anything, you allow yourself to explore and be talented in. Your expression. Wonderful sky blue color here with silver sparkles. The silver sparkle is the Goddess energy, a more feminine form. It allows you to just BE expression. Embody expression. Radiate expression. Demonstrate expression. Infuse any form of expression with love. Call upon the devas of whatever instrument you work with Divine Creativity. Work with the materials. Work with the cells of the materials. And allow them to mix together in a wonderful synthesis of being. Light blue is spinning clockwise, empowered and full of your being.

Take a deep breath, moving up the channel, widening the channel to your third eye. You are becoming more and more psychic and more intuitive in rhythm with your soul development. Allow this area to expand gently and easily. You use guidance for yourself first, and then for others, if that is what you are called on to do. Remembering to balance dreamtime healing with daytime healing. Remembering your first two channels of psychic awareness. Knowing you can develop them. Love them as a gift from Spirit. Whether that be clairsentience, clairvoyance, claircognizance, or clairaudience. All are equal. All are good. Allowing them to open and allow yourself to be in reality at the same time. For as you walk between the two worlds it is very important at this time to be in reality. Beautiful indigo color here connected to the higher realms of consciousness.

Taking a deep breath, moving up the channel, widening the channel coming to the crown chakra. Anchoring in the Christ Consciousness grid energy and bringing it through the crown chakra. This is only the start, allowing the energy to come down through each chakra, all the way down past your feet to your Moment of Self. You know you are connected to Spirit. You know that you are supported. Allow yourself to feel your Higher Self and call it in everyday to be in total alignment with Spirit. Please answer the call, and trust your inner guidance, bringing it here on earth. Know that as you place your hands in prayer position, or in the healing mudra, you can activate the Reiki energy. Feel this energy, however it is for you to perceive it. Allow yourself to heal your entire aura and anchor this healing into infinity. Being in the fullest and best way now.

Taking a deep breath, and allowing the energy to rise up from the earth. The crystalline, the lava, in your energy bodies from the feet to your knees, root sacral, solar plexus, heart, up to the throat, up to your 3rd eye up to your crown. Going beyond and spraying down upon you in a wonderful shower of earth energy. Feel the vital earth energy surrounding your aura and filling it completely. Vibrating in Mother Earth. Being a strong spiritual warrior now. Holding the space for you first and filling yourself completely. You are full of vital earth energy. You are a bright light of manifestation, abundance and vitality. You allow this connection to grow in every day and every way. Surrendering to Spirit and allowing the fullest expression of your life purpose to unfold step by step in truth and love.

As we end this meditation if you are going to sleep, you will drift off protected and healed by the angels and by earth it self. If you are to return back to everyday life, you will have access to this energy by just thinking and activating your key phrase Reiki. Knowing the sooner you ask the sooner you will be surrounded in this beautiful light. I give great thanks to all the Beings of Light who attended this session. In gratefulness and love. Namaste.

Waves of the Mother

The intention for this meditation, Kundalini Reiki Level 2, Waves of the Mother is to allow the listener to connect deep within to the waves of energy directly from the core of mother earth. Begin to feel and radiate these waves integrating them in a very gentle and nurturing manner. This is the feminine energy of the Divine and allows one to become and embody feminine features of the light. Through the regular use of this meditation one can be nurtured, comforted and mothered deep within and without becoming a source of strength and power, a center of light for yourself and others.

So lets begin by just placing your mind, body, spirit, and emotions in alignment and opening to the relaxation from head to toe. Allowing the body to sink deeper and deeper into a space of surrender, into a space of allowing, into a space of receiving. As you breathe, just simply be more and more. Bring your inner vision to a place deep within that is completely dark, completely void, and completely potential. Sheer blackness and sheer promise surrounds you now. Breathe in this energy and allow your being to be restored and renewed easily and effortlessly. Floating in the void. Breathing and being surrounded by darkness. You notice up ahead there's a shimmer of light. You go toward that light with all your heart. The light takes the shape of a beautiful flame. Allow your being to reach and accept this flame, drawing it by intention down to your root chakra and accepting the flame of Kundalini Reiki. Knowing this is your sacred light ceremony. Feeling the strength and thinking to you Kundalini Reiki Meditation at least once per day-everyday.

And now taking your awareness to a place in the core of Mother Earth, renewing your connection to the two frequencies of energies. The first is the crystalline energies-from the crystalline core of earth. The second is the lava energy of earth. Seeing these two frequencies rising up in distinct beams of light at your Moment of Self. Spiraling around each other wrapping and ascending up through your energy fields, all the way through your tap root chakra, through your central energy channel, into your Earth Star chakras. Anchoring at the platform but continuing to evolve upward, twisting in a spiral. Breathing and seeing the spiral of energy now at your feet chakras and knee chakras, up and through your root. Feeling the energy rise through the sacral and solar plexus. Accepting the energy in your heart. Allowing it to flow up into your high heart chakra through the beautiful throat chakra. Up all the way to your 3rd eye and crown. Extending through every level of consciousness up to Spirit. Seeing this spiral as your unique set of DNA. Thinking to yourself DNA Attunement, knowing that your full complement of DNA will be cleansed, cleared, renewed and activated gently and surely through the constant use of this attunement.

Taking a deep breath now and think or say to yourself, Waves of the Mother. Accepting this energy as it enters your field in waves from the Mother Earth. Coming in to surround you and enfold you in beautiful vibration and frequency.

Gentle nurturing earth energy. These beautiful waves will be continuous throughout the meditation.

So now as you receive you bring your awareness to your tap root chakra, a place about 24 " below your feet. Sensing the potential deep within this beautiful rich loam place. See if there are any old contracts here that you have made with others in an unaware or unconscious way. Ask that they are renegotiated or destroyed now, allowing a beautiful strong Archangel named Metatron to come in and clear out this space. He gives you the strength to reshape your life to the full potential to be filled with your goals, opportunities and divine life mission holding it in infinity and sacredness. Allowing it gestate until it wants to be reborn in just the right form.

Taking a deep breath and moving your awareness now to the Earth Star chakras-beautiful little stars about 12 " below your feet. Feel the emerald green light infused here by AA Raphael. You are anchored to earth with Love. Earth is now a very peaceful and wondrous place for you to be. You allow yourself to bring only the best loving nurturing frequencies as AA Michael puts a protective shield around your entire energy field. Keeping out anything that is no longer for your Highest Good. You can still be and see around everything in your life but only that which is for the Highest Good will enter into your sacred energy field. Know this and own this. Feel the emerald light. Feel the connection with beloved AA Michael as your divine protector angel. He will be with you now and always.

Moving your awareness to your feet chakras, a beautiful black color and allow yourself to move on your path with strength and might. We ask for a connection here with the Goddess Kali, a magnificent goddess of death, destruction and might. It is the death of the ego that we are called upon to embrace anytime that you feel you need to let go of something that is no longer for your Highest Good. You do the dance of Kali. By intention making a ball of energy that represents the form that you feel you want to bless and release in the light. Pulling it below your feet and stomping it, just as Kali would, with great might and power. Knowing your prayer will be answered. Feel the confidence in allowing yourself to release as the first step that is needed in order to receive.

Taking a deep breath, moving your awareness now to the movement chakras at your knees. They are a beautiful brown color. We ask for an infusion of citrine crystalline light here that you may move with manifestation power. The citrine ray will allow one to really be conscious and aware of the power of your intention and manifestation consciousness. Call in this ray to surround all your creations, goals, and lists of requests on the New Moon Day. Making sure that the manifestations are moving at the rhythm and alignment of your soul and Divine Will. Writing them down and releasing them to the universe. Seeing the wings of doves here, flapping and moving peacefully in this chakra.

Taking a deep breath and moving your awareness up to your root chakra. This is a sacred place of connection, this foundation here on earth. You allow yourself to connect in the light to great angels, beings, and ascended masters. You bring all of your Healing team now from your crown down now to your root chakra to help you be really functional and strong a source of power in everyday life. You are now a vortex of abundance. You are someone who can clearly and easily manifest what you need to support yourself in life. So allowing yourself to connect with the Divine, Healing team, brothers and sisters of the light, soul family, monad, Spirit at all levels bringing down your chakras and anchoring the light from your heart with this beautiful clear ruby chakra.

Taking a deep breath, moving awareness to the second chakra that sacral chakra, beautiful orange here. You not only have your unity attunement but you allow an overlay of the triple aspect of the Goddess. The innocent child, fertile maiden, and wise crone. Allow your being to sense these energies and to interweave them, into a beautiful unified second chakra. Being in joy as a child, being a creative expression as a maiden, and being a wise teacher as a crone. Accept these gifts. Own them. Be with them. Embody their strength and joy.

Taking a deep breath, bringing your awareness to your solar plexus. Being totally in Divine Will. Allowing the Solar Logos energy to be infused fully here. This is a powerful Being of Light. He is here to keep you and your connection between heaven and earth open. So, just allow this to be opened and to be infused with beautiful energy coming in. Anytime you want to renew and restore, think Solar Logos Attunement. You simply step outside to the sun and allow yourself to bring in the energy through your crown and down into your solar plexus. Totally renewed and restored with this Solar Logos Attunement,

Taking a deep breath, moving into your heart now. This heart energy is now very wide and very expanded. We are going to go ahead and believe and know that our heart energy is now like a satellite dish here. Rounded to receive, be, and transmit your beautiful heart energy out to the entire world. Everyday and in every way you expand your heart chakra holding yourself, family, and all those who you heal and who it is part of your life purpose to be within this beautiful sacred container of your heart. Emerald energy here. Allowing this energy to expand and encompass the entire world. Being love. Receiving loving. Giving love. This is your reality. This is your strength. Accept this in the light.

We now ask for beautiful heart concentrated energy to come in. See Quan Yin, Mother Mary, Lady Theresa holding this space for you. Allowing your being to be nurtured and loved everyday in every way. Bringing it out of into the world with confidence, wisdom, and power. So not only are you balanced in mind body spirit and emotions, but you are also integrated with three-fold flame of love wisdom and power.

Taking a deep breath, bringing your awareness to your soul purpose chakra. Allowing an infusion of light from Beyond the Goddess to come now into this space, opening out this area with the Seven rays of ascension. Allow them to anchor here in a very integrated fashion. Allow them to come down from the sky and up from the earth mixing in your soul purpose chakra. Spreading out in beautiful rays now to all those who you meet. Seeing the various colors, frequencies, strengths of these beautiful rays of creation. For you are Namaste in Love and Light.

Taking a deep breath moving up to your throat chakra now. We are going to ask that your heart energy come up and be anchored permanently in your throat. This very special connection will allow you to speak from your heart. We also ask for an etheric link here. We ask that this very special link from your heart to your throat be empowered with the strength of the Waves of the Mother of Kundalini Reiki Level 2. So each time you speak, your words contain the frequency of these waves. Those listening receive a healing through your words, through your vocal expression. Each time you practice Reiki, or meditation these waves increase in frequency, strength and power. Beautiful light blue here. Beautiful voice and vocal chakra.

Taking a deep breath, moving your awareness to your third eye allowing yourself to explore spirituality, dreamtime healing modalities, and spirit creatively. Activating in this chakra by intention your Ascension Seat Activation Attunement. This activation attunement allows a part of your soul to journey twenty-four hours a day, seven days a week and sits in the ascension seats or etheric places of wisdom in temples through out space and time. Learning, receiving healings, and knowing. So by calling upon this specific attunement, you are enforcing your specific intention to become ascended, to become knowledgeable in the light, and to open fully and completely to your psychic and intuitive gifts. Seeing the indigo blue here. Seeing your strength and power of your womanly rite to healer, visionary and teacher to know.

Breathing and bringing your attention now to your crown chakra. Allowing Sprit to guide you. Taking a deep breath calling forth a beautiful pillar of light to come down and surround your entire being in light. We ask that through this tube of light you receive a beautiful aquamarine shimmer mist that activates your energy to the Goddess. Feel and receive this wonderful infusion now knowing that as you stay clear and connected to the earth, you can anchor this beautiful Goddess energy and become a conduit for Spirit in purity, goodness and light.

Know this and accept this. We like to thank all the Higher Beings of Light who assisted with this healing now. We ask for the Waves of the Mother to be awakened in all. Namaste in Love and Light.

Diamond Energy Completion

The intention of this meditation, Kundalini Reiki Level 3, Diamond Energy Completion, is to allow the listener to receive each time a profound energy clearing using the healing Reiki sequence. In addition, this meditation contains extra attunements that focus on gentle energy integration. The listener is invited to journey to the etheric diamond pyramid to participate fully in a powerful ceremony with ascended master Kuthumi. Through regular use of this recording, one can gain initiatory status into profound wisdom of the soul providing the next steps to complete the sacred life purpose. Intend to co-create with Kuthumi a life balanced in love wisdom and power.

So let's begin. Taking several very deep and cleansing breaths. Filling the belly up with air on the inhale. Intending relaxation for the phsycial body and exhaling. Drawing in the belly, intending to release any tension from head to toe. Inhaling intending peace, focus, and transpersonal awareness from the mind. Exhaling, intending letting go with love and neutrality any distractions. Inhaling intending calm and peaceful emotions coming to still point. Exhaling, intending to release any disruptive emotional processes. Inhaling, intending connection to Higher Self and Spirit awakens the soul. Exhaling separation and limitation.

Resting at still point. Feeling the energies as you put your hand chakras together. First in masculine, active prayer position and thinking the key phrase Reiki. Sensing the energy flow. Exhaling and shifting your hand position to the feminine mudra. Thinking the key phrase, Kundalini Reiki, as the energy flows. Now we will begin breath of fire while shifting our hands in a rhythmic manner as we breathe and run the energy. Breath of fire is quick forceful exhale through the nostrils while pulling in our belly and diaphragm. Think Reiki and breath of fire changing hands masculine. Breath of fire. Feminine. Sky. Earth. Vertical. Horizontal. Crossroads. Moving beyond space and time.

As you continue your fire breathing, visualize yourself sitting in the middle of a barren desert in the middle of two roads. Immense father sky: Limitless mother earth. Feel your Kundalini flame begin to build in your first chakra sensing the energy at the base of the spine wound up in a snake like coil. Breathing out and building. Feeling the energy in your pelvic cavity stronger and stronger as it uncoils and begins to expand up and out, filling the main energy channel to the stomach and abdomen radiant with light. Open and moving up to the heart expanding and strengthening surely and strongly up the back and neck, breathing and building to the head and eyes.

Exhaling, strengthening, blessing the energy with the mantra of power: Sat Nam, Sat Nam, Sat Nam. Up and out the crown, Sat Nam, A myriad of small flames burst from the crown around the body. Visualizing now each flame becoming alive and as you slowly resume your normal, deep breath you allow this state of being to expand further into a fully activated Kundalini flame from root to crown.

Asking now to be connected to the Guardian of the Flame. A Higher Being of Light now comes into the sacred space of the crossroads and infuses each of the flames surrounding you with an aspect of spirit. The flame of the north celebrates your uniqueness, joy and gratitude. The flame of the south releases the old, allowing a feeling of groundedness in stability and structure. The flame of the East allows purification of intrinsic worth opening the heart to unconditional love. The flame of the west infuses a creative reality of truth and intuitive knowing. Other flames that surround you now are justice, truth, freedom, healing, wisdom, maturity, health, creativity, spirituality, service, peace, serenity, harmony, freedom, trust, faith, reconciliation, mercy, forgiveness, love, discernment, knowing, being, power, and glory.

See this ring of fire all around , a radiant fiery stonehedge. Dancing in aliveness energetic full. Each cell in your body responds to this very high frequency shower of electric light. Magnetizing, purifying, and preparing yourself for your journey to meet Kuthumi.

Begin to activate now the Diamond Reiki allowing you to sense the enlightenment this Reiki frequency provides. Breathe and relax. Now activate the Crystalline Reiki. Sensing the next place within your energy field where any crystalline form is dissolved and removed transmuted forever. Taking a deep breath and thinking DNA Reiki. This vibrational essence clears the blueprint of our life. Allowing for the future to be full of health and vitality. Thinking or saying to yourself now Birth Trauma Reiki the energy flows tot he moment of your birth surrounding you as a newborn in light. Seeing yourself in an energetic protective womb until you take your first breath of air. Activating the Location Reiki vibration now. Breathing and asking to see your inner vision what external from of matter needs to released as it may be keeping you from your Highest Good. Feeling lighter as the cords fall away. Breathing into your belly and saying Past Life Reiki. Images, body memories, energetic patterns are blessed with this Reiki surrounding them with light and allowing them to be whisked away from your cellular memories.

Moving toward balance now as you place your fingertips together thinking or saying BALANCE. All of your energy is in alignment. All of your self is purified.

Seeing up ahead a large mountain. This symbolizes your spiritual journey at the very top is a large etheric pyramid of Kuthumi. Begin walking up the mountain now on a path. Each step you take brings you closer to Spirit, higher in the light. Notice the foliage around you. What types of trees are there? What sorts of sounds do you hear? What colors do you see? Stopping for a moment about half way there, turning to your right. At the side of the path please surrender something you have identified as a barrier to your spiritual progress. Take a deep breath exhaling and surrendering now.

Resuming your journey a little lighter now. Walking and breathing totally on your life path and in your power. Pausing for a moment about three quarters of the way there and turning to the left side of the path. Receiving a gift from Spirit. It may be an animal, plant, light or symbol. Accept this gift with great love resuming your journey.

Up ahead is the initiatory Crystalline Pyramid of Kuthumi. Stand at the entrance feeling humbled by the massive structure of light. Enter the great room setting your intention of what you wish to say or have cleared in this experience. Moving inside the pyramid to the place of great light. As you stand in this chamber the planetary energies in accordance with the Language of Light will begin a very gentle energy integration. Close your eyes take a deep breath and receive this gift of Spirit now. As you open yourself further, Kuthumi steps forward from the light standing in front of you. Feel the gratitude, unconditional love, and acceptance as you enter a state of communion with your teacher. He presents to you a beautiful diamond harvested from the very top of the pyramid as you intend or say yes, Kuthumi places this beautiful etheric capstone into your crown chakra.

"Dearest one you are perfect whole and complete in Kundalini Light". He blesses and heals each one of your chakras sending you telepathically the next steps of your life purpose directly into your third eye. Take a deep breath, knowing all you have to do to realize these bits of wisdom are to center breath and know.

Kuthumi also sends to you now the Soul Star Attunement this higher chakra attunement when activated will infuse more of your soul light into your body increasing your light here on earth. He also gives to you the Earth Mother attunement. This provided fast grounding and connection to Mother Earth.

Finally say or think the Life Purpose Attunement, then write down or receive your divinely guided ideas for the future.

Taking a deep breath and thanking Kuthumi, preparing to come back into the now. If you are listening to this meditation before bed you drift off into a restful deep dream state. If you are going to return to the now, know that you have been initiated into the Diamond Energy Completion. Taking a deep breath, wiggling your fingers and toes. Coming back into your body. We would like to thank all the higher beings of light that supported this meditation. Namaste. AHO. Shanti.

Chapter 7

Attunement Information

Kundalini Reiki

All attunements are available through contacting the website: http://www.healingevolvement.com

Kundalini Reiki is a complete and simple healing system that connects you deep within to "Spiritual Warrior Energy". This octave of energy clears very gently but effectively, issues and blocks resulting in an increased flow of vital earth energy. Ascended Master Kuthumi works with you to heal and empower you and your life mission here on earth.

Learning Objectives:

Clearing/widening of the main energy channel
Restructuring of the energy system
Learning powerful healing techniques
Extra attunements
Balancing issues related to manifestation, fatigue abundance.

Massive shifts in life toward higher frequency and life purpose.
Raises the Kundalini Flame
Corrects improper Kundalini awakening.

Kundalini Reiki 1

The first attunement opens the healing channels to allow channeling of Reiki energy. At the same time you are prepared for the Kundalini awakening in Kundalini Reiki 2. The Crown, Heart and hand chakras are opened/strengthened. You are taught to perform a complete healing treatment and to heal remotely from a distance. Kundalini Reiki 1 is energy is more masculine with an emphasis on staying in truth.

Kundalini Reiki 2

All channels are strengthened. Kundalini Awakening -main energy channel opens gently and surely, alighting the Kundalini "fire." Kundalini reaches the Solar Plexus chakra, preparing for the full Kundalini rising in Kundalini Reiki 3. You are also taught a specific meditation. When you perform this meditation, you increase in a short time, the power of the flame in the Kundalini fire/energy. In this way, all the chakras/energy systems are enlightened and a cleansing takes place. Energy is more feminine and allows receptivity, being and radiating. Connects one to the Waves of the Mother. There are also very dynamic teachings and attunements in Level 2 designed to fully integrate the Kundalini experience.

Kundalini Reiki 3

The previous Attunements are strengthened and the Throat, Solar Plexus, Hara and Root Chakras are opened. The Kundalini "fire" is strengthened and reaches up and out of the Crown chakra - full rising of the Kundalini takes place. You are taught to attune Crystals and other objects, so that they act as Reiki channels.

Extra included attunements: 1. Balance All. 2. Diamond Reiki. 3. Crystalline Reiki. 4. DNA Reiki. 5. Birth trauma Reiki. 6. Location Reiki. 7. Past Life Reiki. You are also taught to pass on Kundalini Reiki 1-2-3.

Kundalini Reiki Boosters

Prerequisite: Kundalini Reiki 1-2-3. Each of these Attunements strengthens the previously received attunements: Kundalini Reiki 1-2-3. With each step all chakras, the main energy channel and the channels to the hands are widened and strengthened. After Kundalini Reiki Booster 3, your power to channel Reiki will have been increased approx. 100 percent! There are also very dynamic Oral Teachings, Attunements and Techniques in Level 1 2 3* (these oral teachings will improve, expand, enlarge and refine your subtle bodies) are designed to fully integrate the Kundalini experience. You will also be able to pass on the Kundalini Reiki Booster 1-2-3 Attunements.

Chapter 8

About
the
Author

DIRECTOR OF HEALING EVOLVEMENT

Kala Maitri RN, MSN, PhD is a certified Holistic Nurse and Intuitive Healer dedicated to shining Love and Light for Healing Evolvement. An accomplished author, artist, and speaker, Kala has produced CD's for guided meditation: Vital Earth Energy, Waves of the Mother, Diamond Energy Completion, Inward Lotus, and Indigo Journeys. Currently she is implementing a research study entitled: The Effects of a Distance Reiki Renewal Program in Healing Nurses with Burnout. A member of American Holistic Nurses Association, Sigma Theta Tau Honor's Society, Healing Touch International, International Kundalini Yoga Teacher Association, and National Guild of Hypnotherapists. Heart-Centered in Psychiatric Nursing and Private Practice. Kala teaches fully accreditated programs in Energy Healing, Kundalini Yoga, and Reiki.

Kala Maitri

24 Hour Voicemail: (408) 354-4859

Paypal/ e-mail address: lotusfire@earthlink.net

Website: http://www.healingevolvement.

Inward Lotus Intuitive Healing CD

Relax deeply and go on a guided journey to the healing source, your intuitive soul wisdom. Allow connection and development of your intuitive channels. Receive guidance and energy expansion. Move toward peace and acceptance of self. Open to the full potential of being. Allow the soul's destiny to be realized by activatingeach petal of the inward lotus of your heart

NEW MOON/FULL MOON CEREMONIES

The Full Moon Ceremony will be focused on release, forgiveness, and willingness to let go. Please include a letter of what you are releasing for your Highest Good along with your donation and some tobacco or corn meal.

For the New Moon, the focus will be on abundance, manifestation, and gratitude. Please include a letter of what you are trying to bring into your life for your Highest Good along with your donation and some tobacco or corn meal.

The ceremonies will be ongoing and great way to clear Karma and accept the Divine Birthright of Abundance.

Send your package to:

Kala Maitri
c/o Healing Evolvement

(SEE CURRENT ADDRESS LISTED ON WEBSITE)

TITHES

Please consider making Healing Evolvement a place where you send your spiritual tithe.Tithing is the ancient practice of invoking Divine Abundance through giving10% of your income to a place that spiritually inspires you while healing the earth. Tithing is a channel to demonstrate your confidence in Divine Abundance, your birth rite as a spiritual being. It begets the promise of security, protection, and guidance through a high form of philanthropy. Your support of Healing Evolvment insures the light and love are anchored here on earth.

Chapter 9

Product Information

Kundalini Reiki CDs

VITAL EARTH ENERGY - Level 1

Recorded specifically to heal and balance the opening of your energy system while using the energy of Kundalini Reiki.. Kala focuses on chakra clearing, intuitive attunements, and SPIRITUAL WARRIOR ENERGY.

In addition to the use of the Intuitive Flower Essence Spray, listening to this CD provides stability and calmness to your 30- day clearing period.

Waves of the Mother - Level 2

Experience this comforting energetic experience wash over you as you listen. In Waves of the Mother, Kala continues to facilitate the opening of your energy while linking you to the beauty, power and strength of the Earth. Listen frequently after being attuned to Kundalini Reiki Level 2 and restructure your energy gently and easily. Profound!

Diamond Energy Completion – Level 3

The Level 3 Kundalini Reiki CD that contains a powerful ceremony with Kuthumi in the etheric diamond temple. Allows for the completion of the attunements with gentle energy intergation. Explores the next step of your life purpose. Profound wisdom can be attained.

Kundalini Yoga Session

Kundalini Yoga is the sacred technology that promotes awareness from the inside out. It awakens your being to realize your destiny. It is one of the fastest ways to establish and align the relationshp between body, mind, and the soul. Founded by Yogi Bhajan, PhD, Kundalini Yoga is a the ultimate spiritual path for those who can apply discipline and care to your body.

Builds great radiance and grace through powerful, yet simple yoga asanas, pranayama, chanting and much more.

These sessions often include a personalized yoga set based on your healing needs, handout and/ or tape.

Kala is a certified Kundalini Yoga Teacher by the International Kundalini Yoga Teacher Association (IKYTA) and is listed in their directory at http://www.kundaliniyoga. com/

Love Intuitive Flower Essence Reading

Individually handmade by Kala reading your energy and choosing from over 300 BACH, FES, Star Flower essences, various essential oils, Rose Salt from Peru and many, many secrets. Use frequently to cleanse aura and stabilize the emotional body. Spray 12 in from body to stabilize emotions.

* Clears
* Balances
* Re-aligns
• Clients report the spray to be MAGICAL!

Indigo Journeys

A delightful, magical journey for children of all ages to meet and work with their dolphin and angel helpers. Instills positive statements while teaches basic guided meditation. Through powerful healing intention and REIKI, the vocals provide soothing energy and clearing using light and love.

About The Author

Kala Maitri RN, MSN, PhD is a certified Holistic Nurse and Intuitive Healer dedicated to shining Love and Light for Healing Evolvement. An accomplished author, artist, and speaker, Kala has produced CD's for guided meditation: Vital Earth Energy, Waves of the Mother, Diamond Energy Completion, Inward Lotus, and Indigo Journeys. Currently she is implementing a research study entitled: The Effects of a Distance Reiki Renewal Program in Healing Nurses with Burnout. A member of American Holistic Nurses Association, Sigma Theta Tau Honor' Society, Healing Touch International, International Kundalini Yoga Teacher Association, and National Guild of Hypnotherapists. Heart-Centered in Psychiatric Nursing and Private Practice. Kala teaches fully accreditated programs in Energy Healing, Kundalini Yoga, and Reiki.

Printed in the United Kingdom
by Lightning Source UK Ltd.
119896UK00001B/169